White Lies

White Lies

My Personal Struggle with Weight

Cynthia J. Privette

iUniverse, Inc.
New York Lincoln Shanghai

White Lies
My Personal Struggle with Weight

Copyright © 2007 by Cynthia J. Privette

iUniverse books may be ordered through booksellers or by contacting:

iUniverse
2021 Pine Lake Road, Suite 100
Lincoln, NE 68512
www.iuniverse.com
1-800-Authors (1-800-288-4677)

ISBN: 978-0-595-43533-3 (pbk)
ISBN: 978-0-595-87860-4 (ebk)

Printed in the United States of America

To all the beautiful young people I see out there every day who have a weight problem and don't understand why.

Contents

Preface

This book is my story, and it is based solely on my own personal experiences.

I am a fifty-two-year-old woman who can honestly say I've spent the last thirty-three years of my life fighting my weight. This has been an all-consuming goal. My hobbies included learning the newest recipes from the latest health guru and reading up on the latest fad diet. I certainly tried all the new diet clinics, not to mention the most recent exercise craze. My dear husband has been exasperated with me so many times, I should have dedicated this book to him for putting up with me all these years.

When I was young girl in school, we used to hear that the human race might someday colonize space, and I remember thinking how wonderful and exciting that would be. And I'm *still* waiting. Then I always thought that in this computerized space age of ours, those super-smart scientists would finally invent a pill that would allow us to eat all the food we wanted and not get fat. I'm still waiting on that one, too. I've been confined in a self-inflicted prison for the last thirty-three years, desperately searching for a way out. And finally, I have learned that it is the knowledge of the truth that has set me free.

I'm so thankful I finally listened to Jesus. It is my sincere hope that all who read this will be helped and encouraged in some way. At the end of this book I give you a scripture the Lord gave to me after much prayer and fasting. It is both a promise and a warning, for those of you who understand it: *you can finally be free.*

Caution: Never attempt this or any weight-loss program without approval from your physician.

Chapter 1

Is This You?

Who Am I and What Do I Know?

As I describe myself, ask yourself, is this me? For most of my adult life I've struggled with a weight problem. I've tried every diet from A to Z, the low-fat, non-fat, low-carb, boiled-egg, grapefruit, tuna-fish diets, shakes and pills (lots of pills), and so on, and so forth. You get the idea.

I work in an office all day while sitting at a desk, which is obviously not very physical, and up until a year ago, I was *still* trying and trying and trying. But strangely, no matter what I did, instead of getting ahead, I just kept regaining the weight over and over again, plus some extra! I was a career yo-yo dieter, with four sizes of clothes in my closet. I was in deep and sinking fast, and I felt like giving up. What was the answer?

All I wanted to do after working all day was to go through a fast-food drive-through for a hamburger or a pizza, then go straight home, eat of course, then sit down or in many cases, lie down for the evening. My energy level was rock-bottom. I felt absolutely helpless and absolutely hopeless.

I can literally gain pounds in a day. You hear people say, "You didn't gain this weight overnight, and you're not going to lose it overnight." Well that did not apply to me. I could totally blow my diet in a meal and destroy it in one day, and then it might take me weeks to get back to where I was. It also became progressively more difficult the older I became. I had lost interest in the smallest pleasures in life, I didn't want to go out in public because I looked so bad, I didn't have the energy to fix up my house, and I didn't feel like doing any yard work. The only reason I mustered up the energy to go to work every day was because I like to *eat* so much—a catch-22.

Are You Ready?

I mean are you *really* ready? I was sick and tired of being sick and tired. Are you? I had high cholesterol—it was 314 total to be exact. For those of you who don't know how bad that is, it's never supposed to be over 200. A few weeks ago after my last physical, the nurse said, "Your cholesterol is now 174." I was very happy to hear that!

My energy had been nonexistent. I didn't look good, and I didn't feel good. I had turned into a terrible wife, a mediocre housekeeper, and a fast-food junkie. I wasn't even a good friend, because I didn't feel like getting out, so I was always making excuses not to do something. It seemed life was passing me by. I was desperately sure that it was my fault, but I didn't know what to do anymore. I was finally at my wits' end ... finally *done*.

Chapter 2

A Change of Heart

My Dedication

This book is dedicated to all the beautiful young people I see out there all the time who are buried beneath a layer of fat and don't understand why. Kids today are born into a sedentary, high-fat lifestyle, very unlike the one I lived in fifty years ago. The CDC reports that children born in the year 2000 have a fifty-fifty chance of developing heart disease and that type 2 diabetes is now being found in teens, whereas it used to be diagnosed mainly in the fifty and over crowd—both very alarming statistics.

Obesity has become a *major* problem in this country, not only because people are increasingly out of shape, but because of the life-threatening diseases stemming from it. There is a sweeping epidemic of high blood pressure, heart disease, cancer, diabetes, stroke, and high cholesterol in this country. Recent studies show that three quarters of Americans are overweight, with half of that number falling in the "obese" category. My husband and I agreed that when we were in school during the sixties, we might have had one classmate who everyone called the "fat kid." Being overweight was the exception then, certainly not the rule. But something has happened today. It's happened to me, it's happening in our schools, and it's happening to the young and old alike. I recently attended a church social with a group of women of varying ages, from teenagers to elderly, and of that group, only three were remotely in shape. I keep seeing this same scenario everywhere I go.

Point? *America is fat and getting fatter.*

Why?

A lot of people say Americans have drastically changed their lifestyles in the last thirty years. For instance, we drive everywhere we go, we sit at a computer all day, we play computer games instead of going to the gym, we don't take the stairs, we all use the elevator ... I could go on and on.

There's also been a big change in our schools' physical education programs. We once had to attend gym class every day. It was not optional. But these days kids might go once a week. It's true that modern technology hasn't made it any easier for us to be as physically fit as we could be—but I believe that's a very small part of our overall problem. It's status quo everywhere you go; people say the same things over and over again:

1.   Drink eight glasses of water a day.

2.   Take the stairs instead of the elevator.

3.   Limit your fat intake.

4.   Count your calories.

5.   Don't eat too much salt.

6.   Eat green vegetables, but potatoes are bad.

7.   Go for high protein and low carbohydrates!

8.   Eat fruits before 2:00 PM.

9.   Exercise at least three times weekly.

But do you remember what I told you? I've already tried all this stuff over and over again, and the second I attempt to live outside the box, *bam*, the box falls on my head—I mean, my fat head!

When I wasn't getting the proper nutrition, I had no energy, I wasn't in a good mood, my nerves were out of whack, and I couldn't even think straight. Even if I did lose a little weight, who wants to be around someone like that? I was desperate, helpless, hopeless, and almost lifeless. I practically had no life, and I mean no life—read into that what you will. So what's wrong with those ideas?

First of all, there's water: if I drank water all day long, I wouldn't have time to do my job, because I'd spend my day in the bathroom.

Secondly, on these diets where you eliminate whole food groups, it's no wonder you eventually lose it, freak out, and gain all the weight back (and then some).

As for exercise, remember I work at my job eight to ten hours a day, and the *last* thing I feel like doing at the end of a long day is going to the gym or getting on a treadmill.

And diets: the popular diets out there look to me like Tolstoy's *War and Peace*—they're page after page of dos and don'ts and philosophies of every kind. The recipes have ingredients I've never even heard of, and there's always the time issue—it takes *time* to shop for those ingredients, and oh yeah, money to buy all that expensive stuff. And then you have to come home and prepare it, whew! Well there's my exercise!

What's Wrong with "Just Exercise"?

Let me say this before I go any further—been there and done that. Don't work. I'm basically lazy. I really hate exercise. Ironically when I do it, I can see an almost immediate difference, and I actually do feel better. But all that aside, I really hate exercise. When I made myself jog (many years ago), I would be so ill and so mean while I was running that I'd actually imagine all the terrible things I'd do to a mugger if he accosted me.

I can't tell you how many overweight people I know who are industrious. Next to them, I'm a lazy slob. My sister (like myself) has had a weight problem most of her life, but that girl is a ball of fire! I've met many other people just like her, which proves you can be an energetic, hard-working individual and still be overweight. How many skinny lazy people do I know? Quite a few, actually.

Exercise alone won't do it; you must reduce your calories and eat correctly. Now, here's the point of saying all this: yes, exercise is good for you.

Yes, you should do it. Yes, it is helpful in weight control and staying in shape. But ... *it's what we eat that's killing us!*

Even the laziest of us move enough to keep from dying. Neglecting to do fifty sit-ups a day probably won't do you in, but daily donuts with biscuits and gravy will ... fast.

Domino Effect

My mother had always been a tall, slim, very energetic person. She appeared to be the picture of health, and she always looked younger than her years. People always thought we were sisters instead of mother and daughter. When Mama was in her fifties, she started to experience fractures at the least little thing. Once after her nephew gave her a big hug, she had broken ribs. I really didn't know anything about osteoporosis back then, but she was diagnosed with it shortly afterward. In a few short years she lost almost five inches in her height. During this time, she suffered a stroke, and although it was a bad one, by the grace of God she wasn't paralyzed. And then not long after that she suffered a heart attack. One thing seemed to lead to another. All this started to happen when she was at a relatively young age. Thankfully, these days, hospice (which is such a wonderful program) comes in to take care of her. I can't tell you why any of this happened as it did, because I'm not a doctor. But I personally believe her diet left a lot to be desired. Every day of her life, several times a day she would eat homemade biscuits made with white flour and lots of lard, and she'd make gravy or pour white sugar and butter on them. Then she'd take the leftover biscuits and make bread pudding with more white sugar for dessert. She'd often add flour to her vegetables and say she was "putting thickening in them." But it's called *thickening* for a reason, folks. It thickens the foods all right but it does the same thing to our bodies! Another favorite dessert of hers was rice pudding made with white rice and lots of sugar (of course). And her favorite daily drink was iced tea with lots of sugar. Flour, flour, flour, and sugar, sugar, sugar, and when we ate rice, it was white, white, white. Oh my!

Chapter 3

The Diet

No White Flour, No White Sugar, No White Rice

I say on the cover of this book that God gave me two principles to get slim and stay slim the rest of my life. The next two rules you must remember are the principles that I explain in detail throughout the book.

This is the number-one rule you must remember: no white flour, no white sugar, and no white rice.

The number-two rule you must remember is what you should eat every day until you reach your goal weight.

These two things are all important, but I make them easy to remember (which is what I like). Also it's something easy to live with and very easy to do (again, what I like).

And that's it.

The List

Every day, eat the listed serving sizes of all items below except vegetables, which are unlimited.

1. **2 proteins (Note: men add 1 protein a day)**

2. **1 potato**

3. **2 fruits**

4. **1 dairy**

5. **2 whole-wheat breads**

6. **1 deliberate fat**

7. **Unlimited green/salad vegetables**

8. **Beverages you like (sugar-free of course)**

Then What?

When you lose the weight you want, add serving sizes of beans, corn, and nuts to your diet to maintain. You will eat every day off the following list:

1. **What you want.**

2. **When you want it**

3. **How you want it.**

Don't count calories. All you need to do is remember your two rules. And don't forget to eat *serving sizes* of everything except vegetables.

Proteins (2) Can be steak, chicken, fish, eggs, pork, turkey, etc.

Potato (1) Eat every day, mashed, baked, boiled, fried w/o fat unless this is where you use your *deliberate fat.*

Dairy (1) Eat one a day—can be a glass of skim milk, fat-free cheese, fat-free cottage cheese, or fat-free yogurt.

Fat (1) Can be butter on a potato, dressing on a salad, cheese on a whole-wheat pizza, etc.

Breads (2) Must be whole wheat, can be whole-wheat pancakes, slices of bread, whole-wheat pizza, bagels, etc.

Fruits (2) All fruits—mixed tropical fruit, melons, etc.

Greens/salad vegetables (unlimited) Green beans, spinach, zucchini, etc. No limits.

Remember: You will add beans, corn, and nuts when you reach your goal.

Tips

*Spread your proteins and dairy throughout the day so that you won't feel famished.

*If your stomach feels like it has a hole in it (maybe before bedtime, for example, if you had an early dinner), take a few drinks of skim milk, which will also help you sleep.

*Always eat a *variety* of foods in *all* food groups. This will keep you healthy and feeling good.

*Take a good daily vitamin supplement. I take one every day.

*About that water: Water is good for you, so drink it when you're thirsty. A good rule of thumb is to drink one glass first thing in the morning before you do anything else. My husband has done this for years, and he claims to never have problems with being irregular or dehydrated. But also drink stuff you like throughout the day, such as coffee, tea, soft drinks, lemonade, etc. (sugar-free, of course).

*About that exercise: As you lose weight, your energy level will pick up anyway, but it doesn't hurt to walk a little more, and if you have a stair-stepper or treadmill that you currently use as a clothes hanger, clean it off and use it when you feel like it.

Be Creative!

Haven't we all been pretty creative when fixing great food to eat? I cannot be adamant enough—*don't stop now!* It is more important than ever to use a little imagination so you can eat really good, great-tasting, and nutritious foods that will serve you well the rest of your life.

Remember to eat everything on the list every day in serving sizes (your choice). Never touch the forbidden white foods. Add beans, corn, and nuts in serving sizes to your diet after you reach your desired weight. These foods are nutritious but starchy and high in calories, and nuts are also high in fat.

Chapter 4

Set the Stage

Preparation, Preparation, Preparation

There are four cornerstones of success for any diet plan. The first is **motivation**—you must be motivated to want to lose weight. Maybe you want to live long enough to see your grandchildren go to college, maybe you want to have a more active lifestyle, or maybe you've always dreamed of wearing a size 10.

The second is **dedication**—you must be dedicated to sticking with a new lifestyle, and this means commitment. The third is **education**—this means educating yourself continually on good carbs, bad fats, the most nutritious foods, and so forth. Always be in the know. The fourth is **preparation**—and it is by far the most important, because it is the one that can sink you *fast*. I will go so far as to say the reason most food addicts like myself have failed so miserably so many times was the lack of preparation.

I watch a lot of survival shows and documentaries, and I notice the same thing time after time when the adventurers get lost in the wilderness or stranded on a mountaintop or lost at sea. They're usually never *totally* prepared for what they encounter. Most of them are very motivated (gung-ho in fact), and they're dedicated to getting out of their situation. Many of them are also athletes or outdoorsmen—in other words, they're very educated about their surroundings. But too often they make critical mistakes: They don't tell anyone which wilderness they're hiking into, and then when they get hurt, they have to wait for days before anyone can find them. They get caught in a blizzard without the proper attire or equipment. Or they don't pack adequate amounts of water when traveling through a desert. All of these scenarios are akin to someone handing a carpenter a pocketknife and telling him to build a mall. Keep in mind, he has motivation, dedication, and education—but he what he needs are cranes, dump trucks, and crews. He needs *preparation*, and that pocketknife won't cut it! The same thing is true with your diet: if you aren't prepared in *every situation*, you'll get hungry and weak, and you'll ultimately eat the wrong things because they are most readily available and because you are not prepared!

I recently took a class in a neighboring city. I knew that hotel would serve breads and pastries made with white flour and white sugar, and I was right. But because I knew to be prepared, I had carried a large whole wheat bagel and a banana with me. So I ate their ham on my bagel and instead of cake, I ate my fruit.

Preparation, preparation, preparation. I cannot stress this enough. It will make you or break you!

The Mental Factor

If preparation is the number one thing to derail your diet, then your mental state certainly is number two. Mood swings, depression, and stress are three great enemies that can and will sabotage your diet. You hear more about stress today than ever before, because everybody is trying to burn the candle at both ends, especially us women. We usually work outside the home—which can be an aggravation itself—but on top of our jobs, we still have housework, shopping, cooking, committees, and a host of other things consuming our time. The workload is doubled if you are a woman with small children, and for those of us in the over-fifty crowd, we also have to negotiate the topsy-turvy world of hormones. And then there are those of us subjected to negative people, who are always belittling, demeaning, and criticizing us. (An unfortunate few are married to these people.) If you're a young woman with a boyfriend who's always telling you how fat and unattractive you are—dump him! Trust me, you can do better; and before long, baby, you'll be able to do much better. If you have a so-called friend who's always insulting you in an off-handed sort of way—get rid of her! The only one that kind of friend loves is the one he or she sees in the mirror. If someone discouraged you as a child—get over it! Those days are gone. Don't be a prisoner of the past. Say goodbye to it.

The same way you would protect your physical body from harm in an attack is the way you need to protect your mind and emotions from negative outside influences. Surround yourself with positive things and positive people.

Just remember: a positive, goal-oriented attitude is priceless in every way.

Chapter 5

To the Point

Realistically Speaking ...

There are statistics from different regions of the world whose inhabitants have reported life expectancies that far exceed our own. Some may consume particular nutrients in their diets (available only in their area of course), and others live at high altitudes, giving them superior respiratory systems. Still others go to bed at sundown and get many more precious hours of sleep than the rest of us. And finally, there are people in some countries who are practically never diagnosed with colon cancer, heart disease, or high blood pressure. Many experts promote these countries' lifestyles as "the way" to good health and long life.

The primary audience I'm addressing, however, is the one I'm most familiar with, and that is those of us who live mostly sedentary, fast-food lifestyles. When is the last time any of us ate an eggplant cooked in extra virgin olive oil with a side hunk of hunza bread on the island of Crete? Anyone ...?

The fact is that many people invest their time and money in *unrealistic* weight-loss programs that call for food they don't eat, can't find, or don't even recognize. This is like spending your money on those irresistibly fancy rhinestone-laden party clothes and spike-heeled shoes that, in reality, you'll never have an appropriate opportunity to wear. In like manner, too many people buy into diets that seem stylish but are, in the reality of the daily grind, impractical. Or they might buy expensive prepackaged food but then still have to buy fresh fruits and vegetables to add to it. Then they purchase expensive exercise equipment and tapes for exercises they may not even be able to do. I tried an exercise program recently, and I could never make it out of the beginner's stage, because as the program advanced, the extreme movements put you in such configurations, a contortionist couldn't get out of them. Guess how long I stuck with that one?

In truth, you can lose weight on almost any diet that restricts your calorie intake. But the question you have to answer is this:

Is this diet or fitness program something I can realistically live with _every day_, based on my lifestyle, physical ability, environment, and the food available in my area?

Catch Phrases

Several years ago you'd hear the popular catch phrases, "fat makes you fat" and "a calorie is a calorie is a calorie …"—both of which (by themselves) have deceptive connotations. Like everyone else, I tried the totally fat-free program, but I quickly realized that I'd never been so miserable or mean in my life as I was on that diet. My nerves went berserk, and I didn't even lose _that_ much weight. But one good thing came out of all that hoopla—the market responded in a big way to the battle cry. Nowadays you can buy almost anything fat free, but unfortunately people have a tendency to think fat free is also calorie free—_not true_. But regardless, fat calories are like any other calories in that if you don't burn them off, your body will store them as fat—it just doesn't have to go to any trouble to convert it to fat because it's _already_ fat. Bottom line is this: if you eat too many calories _of any kind_, and you don't burn them off, you'll gain weight. As I said before, some fat is good for you, but try to avoid excess animal fats as much as possible and choose vegetable oils instead.

To say a calorie is a calorie is calorie implies you can drink a liter of cola or eat a sandwich with an equivalent number of calories and be just as well off. But nothing could be farther from the truth. When consuming any kind of calories, you should always be after _nutrition_. Some calories are empty: they do absolutely nothing for your body, health, mind, nerves, or looks. They're just something else for you to burn off to keep from getting fat without offering you anything in return.

The third catch phrase I'd hear was "the clothes make the woman." Do you know what I'd have if I put a pink tutu on a pig? The answer is: a pig with a pink tutu on it. When I would be thin (for the moment), almost anything could look reasonably decent on me, but when I was fat, almost nothing, and I mean nothing, looked good on me. If you put a bag over Sophia Loren's head, the part of her you *could* see would make you *want* to see the rest. You know what I mean?

Addiction

My only son passed away a while back. He had struggled with drug addiction over the years. He had finally met the girl of his dreams, and he was looking forward to a bright future. He would pull himself up time and time again, go through rehab, and get back to work and then suddenly he'd lose the fight and fall back into drugs. In a way I understand, and under those very difficult circumstances, I guess he put up a pretty good fight after all.

God bless my dear mother, she always meant well when she'd say things like, "Just eat *one* piece of cake; it won't hurt you." But she didn't understand I couldn't eat just *one* of anything! On one occasion I was telling my husband how people would say to me, "Oh I can't eat that piece of candy, it's almost lunchtime," or "I *would* have a slice of pie, but it would ruin my appetite." And my favorite is "You know I got so busy today, I forgot to eat." (How could you *possibly* forget to eat?) I asked him what these things meant. He said, "A hog like you would never understand."

I saw a television show recently about people who had lost tremendous amounts of weight—one man had even lost over 300 pounds, which is truly amazing. He and others like him were motivated by circumstances in their lives to get the weight off. I am a self-proclaimed food addict, and I know there are others out there just like me. I want to comment on what I feel is the biggest difference between food addicts and other kinds of overeaters. Some people gain weight as the decades pass, not necessarily because they eat any differently, but because their metabolism slows down or because they're not as active as they once were. Then there are people who do eat a lot—maybe overeating out of boredom, or maybe overeating because they do not have access to nutritious foods all the time. Food addicts on the other hand are much like drug addicts: they want to quit, but they can't. They will do very extreme things when it comes to food: they will lie, cheat, hide food, destroy evidence of it, hoard it, or steal it (yes, steal it). They hide where no one will see them eat all this food, and then they lie about it. They feel guilty and terrible and ashamed and out of control, because they *are* out of control! We food addicts don't always need to lose 300 pounds, but we keep losing and regaining the same 50-plus pounds over and over and over again, and we keep losing ground. Meanwhile, the only thing that's spiraling downward is our health and our morale. If we have a cake in the freezer, we don't wait for it to thaw; we eat it frozen! I've heard so many people say they were out of control. Well, meet the woman who could have coined that phrase and whose picture would appear by the definition if it were in the dictionary.

Chapter 6

Little Tales of Woe

Donut Story

I'd just come from a crusade in Durham, North Carolina, and I was on my way home at about one in the morning. I had stopped at a drive-in window to get two dozen donuts, which were drenched in glaze and still warm, fresh from the oven. I ate one, then another, and another. I reached over and realized I had eaten both boxes in just a few minutes. I don't know if there's such a thing as a sugar coma, but if there is, I don't know why I didn't go into one. I freaked out and drove to a deserted area, jumped out of the car, and threw the empty boxes down an embankment. I felt like someone disposing of a body! Does that sound like someone in control to you?

The Candy Bars

I always hoarded food when we traveled anywhere near or far. I usually would carry drinks, candy, pastries, and my over-the-counter, caffeine-laden drugs (you know, in case I got lost in the wilderness or something).

On our first cruise, I had a few things stashed away but ran out before we got to Nassau, Bahamas. The ship sold my favorite soda beverage, but they wanted an arm and a leg for it (it was considered a bar drink), and even I wasn't going to pay that price if I could help it. So after docking, I immediately got off the ship, ran past everyone, and hired the fastest horse and buggy available to find my soda in town. Every store we went to didn't have my usual junk food or drinks. *I felt so helpless.* Who would ever think about stashing food on a cruise ship? They're known for practically feeding you to death. But they didn't serve what I wanted!

When we arrived in Newport, I saw a candy machine (be still my heart) and ran over and immediately bought six candy bars. Then I sat down and ate them all at once. I remember I didn't want much supper on board that night. Maybe that's what people mean when they say, "I don't want that candy, it will ruin my dinner"!

How could something I want ruin something else I want?

After arriving back in Key West Florida, I looked around at all the clean nice shops with tons of my goodies at each checkout in every store. I said "Oh America, America!" I suddenly realized I wouldn't last 3 minutes in a wilderness.

Stretch Pants Incident

Stretch polyester pants are what I've worn since I was a teenager. People would always say, "Why don't you wear jeans like all the other girls?" I would answer by explaining how comfortable those stretch pants were, but I really wore them because they were so forgiving as my weight went up and down (mostly up) through the years. One of my great goals was to finally be able to wear jeans like everyone else, and oh yes, a swimming suit!

My height is under five foot four, so at 195 pounds, my stretch pants were being asked to do *a lot*. I usually wore a big shirt to come down over my hip area, but on one particular day, I discovered that I needed a *longer* shirt.

I had sat down abruptly at my desk when I heard a loud rip. I quickly stood up and felt an immediate draft. I thought, *Oh no, oh no!* Slowly I felt the back of my pants, only to find that the whole seat had ripped out! I work in a maintenance shop filled with men, and the nearest exit to my car was a walk through the entire plant with people everywhere. Luckily I kept a big old shirt hanging on a hook by the door; I immediately grabbed it, wrapped it around me, and slowly started heading for the door. But I was in a panic and forgot my badge which opens the gate to get out. I was moving very slowly so that no one would see my underwear as I walked. At the gate, I frantically punched the button so security would let me out, but they didn't see me. And who should pull up behind me but our plant manager? He was waving for me to get out of my car and get his badge so we both could get out—but I pretended not to see him. The guard finally saw me … thank God.

I would never admit to wearing anything larger than a size 12 (talk about fantasy land), even though it might be stretched out to a size 2X—call it vanity, stupidity, or whatever. My usually trustworthy pants were indeed labeled size 12 on the inside tag, and all those years I never abandoned them. But on this particular day, *they* abandoned *me*. After this incident, I did what every conscientious woman would do—I went on another fad diet!

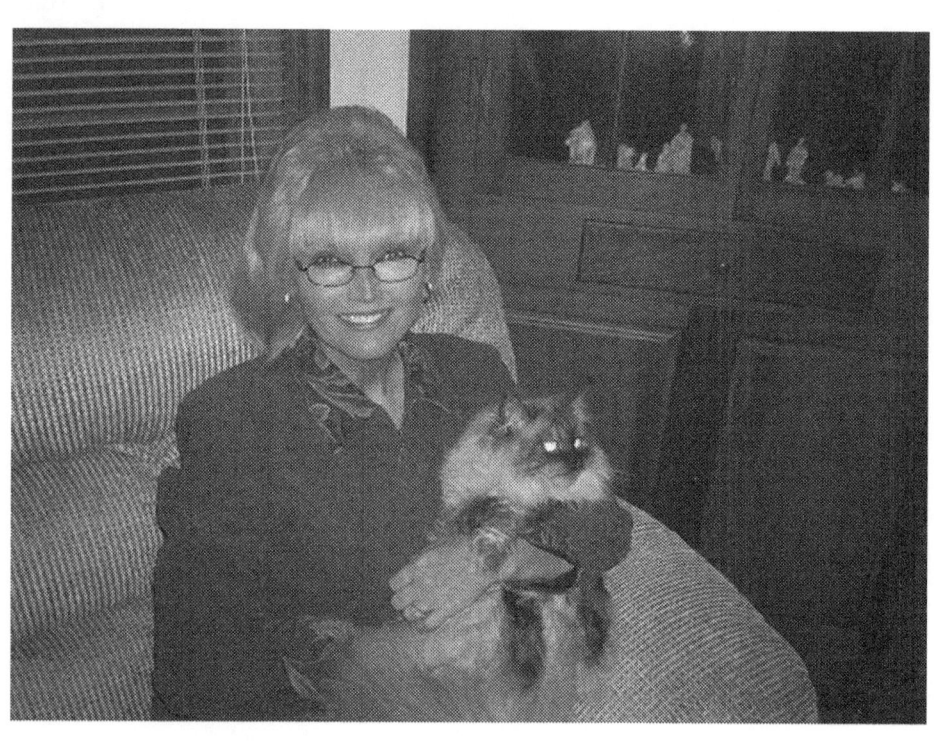

Chapter 7

State of Mind

Regular, Normal, and "a little something"

"Regular" and "normal" were the two most overused and least understood words in my vocabulary. I had a language all my own. I could never understand why I was such a mess. When I would finally break and eat three chili cheeseburgers with fries and a chocolate shake (it was probably much worse than that), I would always look at someone thin (of course) and say, "But I'm only eating *regular* food like *normal* people do."

I remember on one morning, I had really bad heartburn (and oh yeah, I had gotten up to taking a whole box of antacid a day). I told my friend about it, and she wanted to know what I had eaten the night before. I said, "*A little something*, I believe it was two pieces of Sicilian pizza." She looked at me in shock; she said, "Cynthia, two pieces of pizza is *not* a little something; a little something is more like a few bites of pudding." I wouldn't have known "regular" or "normal" if they bit me in the butt! And you know what I thought "a little something" was.

Excuses

There was no such thing as having a piece of birthday cake at someone's party for me, because I would go into a tailspin for weeks, maybe even months. Then I'd tell myself I had to be "in the mood" to start my diet again. Of course I'd have excuses like "It's my birthday" or "It's Christmas," or "We're on vacation, and it's our anniversary for crying out loud—of course I should be able to be a pig if I want, and besides I'm not in the *mood* to diet!"

The excuses for my weight included things like, "I have big bones," "I'm so short, I just look heavier," "That darn cleaner is shrinking my clothes," and my all-time favorite, "I have a slow-burning metabolism." I guess it was slow—it should have been non-existent after I drowned it in white poison for thirty years! But what I've learned is this: when fed the right foods, after all the abuse I've put it through, and even at fifty-two years of age, my body has a butt-kicking metabolism!

I asked the Lord one day if I couldn't eat something "good" on special occasions (you food addicts know what I mean), and in the spirit He gave me a resounding *No*. I suppose that would be like someone who smokes cigarettes with lung cancer saying, "Well can't I smoke just *one* on my birthday or New Years Day?" What would we be celebrating anyway—disease and addiction? The answer is no.

Excuses? I had a million of them.

Never on Sunday

I could never bring myself to start a diet on any day but Monday. The weekend was definitely out, because that was my downtime. Monday was the first day of the work week, and anyway it already required a lot of discipline. So my strategy was to start a new diet program on a Monday, and if for any reason I blew it during the week, I'd say, "Well, I've already messed up, so I may as well eat. I'll start again next, what ... Sunday? No." Never on Sunday. But next Monday (if I was in the mood). And so it went for thirty-three years ...

Chapter 8

A Strategy

What Happened?

Two years ago I went to see my doctor. I hadn't seen her in a while, so I was stunned to see her so thin. I almost didn't recognize her at all, because her appearance had changed so dramatically. When I ask her what she'd done, she briefly described her diet, and all I can fully remember is how she stressed not eating white flour, white sugar, and white rice. She said you could eat whole-wheat products or brown rice instead.

Although I was terribly impressed, I guess at this point, I still wasn't *ready*. Then something else happened. One day an entertainer I like very much was talking about making chocolate-chip cookies (my favorite). And she said something I'll never forget. She said yes how much fun it was to make these cookies for the holidays, but she said that she didn't eat stuff like that anymore. I thought, *Anymore, like never?* I always thought that once you found "the answer," somewhere, somehow you could finally go back and eat chocolate-chip cookies! I mean *never?* And as unfathomable as that was to me, somehow it stuck. I didn't forget what she said because she obviously knew something I certainly did not. Unfortunately I kept trying this diet and that diet. Did I mention I also spent a small fortune on diet-related products?

Success

Other people seemed to achieve success, but as odd as it might sound, I still had to (in a sense) do it my way.

I prayed. I asked God to help me. He's really the one who caused me to remember those two things. You might say, well Cynthia, you've been a Christian a long time … why now? Or why did you finally listen to the Lord *now*? Remember what I said? You have to be *ready* to listen. I always thought the most fatal thing someone can think. I thought, *I can handle it.* (Famous last words.)

When thinking about the types of foods I felt satisfied eating every day, surprisingly the things I really liked to eat, I can eat—potatoes for one thing. Being from the South, I ate some kind of potato almost every day of my life. Potatoes generally take a bad rap in diets, not because they're bad for you—on the contrary, they're actually very nutritious—but because they're high in calories. But you need energy, and this great vegetable's benefits far outweigh the bad. Fat has also been labeled public enemy number one on many diet plans, however you actually need *some* fat to keep you healthy, just not large amounts. Bread, I love bread, and I can have it, and all fruits, and all meats.

The Lord brought me back to basics—eating from all of the food groups daily and omitting as much processed food as possible.

Saying Too Much

There's such a thing as saying too much. Some diet plans tell you exactly what to eat, when to eat it, how to eat it, how to cook it … you may even have to weigh it. You're so hemmed in, there's no joy whatsoever in eating. Your whole life is consumed with an unpleasant task.

You only have to remember the two principles in this book:

> No white flour, no white sugar, and no white rice.
> Eat foods off the list every day.

Use spices, be creative in preparing your foods, eat when you're hungry, and enjoy life. I love simplicity, and after thirty years of the run-around, I don't want to have to remember a lot of rules and regulations. If I want the answer to something, I don't want a lengthy instruction manual. I just want *the answer*.

So many foods are "empty" foods, filled with calories but very little or no nutrition. Ask yourself:

1. What is it that's robbing my health, my looks, my vigor, my life?

2. Do I intend to let this go on? Am I going to continue down this self-destructive road?

3. Are the chocolate-chip cookies *so important?*

4. Can't I go home again? Can't I?

We somehow think we can go back to the way we were and do the things we used to do. But that's like saying we're going to jump back into that same fire and not get burned again. A fire is still a fire, though, and you're still you. We can no longer let it destroy us, but instead find a way to make it work for us.

Chapter 9

A New Way of Thinking

Addressing a Former Statement

Remember how I said something was happening to us as a society? America is fat and getting fatter with no prejudice at all between young or old, black or white, rich or poor. I conclude that it certainly is a combination of bad habits in our overall lifestyle as a society. But there are wrong, wrong, wrong food choices on every street corner. Just look around. And in almost every case, there are no alternative choices to make in breads or sugary treats or the rice prepared in these foods.

If there is one thing I'd like to see change in this country, it would be the choices in all restaurants, including pizza parlors and fast-food joints. When you pull up to a window, they should say, "Whole wheat or white with that?"

Balance and Moderation

What then makes this diet different from the others? Well for one thing, it addresses fidelity, and I've never come across another diet plan that stresses this important principle. Secondly you have to realize this is a life-changing endeavor—there's no going back. The diet itself is based solely on the two principles that the Lord gave me—first, eliminating the foods that were destroying my health and weight issues; and secondly, eating a balanced, nutritious diet in moderation every day. Actually you have to relearn how to eat, and after fifty-two years, I learned to eat again. You might say I had to start from scratch, really. In reality you can lose weight on almost any diet—but can you keep it off? And is the diet plan nutritionally sound?

Many times, in a mad rush to get your weight down (I know all about this), you will sacrifice nutrition, which in the long run will do more harm than good. Keep in mind what I said about eliminating food groups. Your body will eventually rebel, because it lacks nourishment, and you will begin to eat the wrong things again as well as overeat again. Some will think if they skip a food today and another one tomorrow they'll lose weight faster, but in reality (again), what they're doing is setting themselves up for failure. Let me reiterate the importance of *balanced daily nutrition*. You need a strong mind and body to be able to make sound, rational decisions and to remember the things you need to remember. Then you have to have the energy to get it all done.

There are no shortcuts to true and lasting success!

Unfortunately, statistics still show that most people who've lost weight on various diet plans will regain their weight. So don't be a statistic.

Scales

I'd like a nickel for every day of my life that was absolutely ruined by getting on my bathroom scale. I look back and see how truly ridiculous that was. So let me say this first: get rid of those scales!

Your body is *always* in the process of repair, regeneration, and overall maintenance, using whatever means necessary for optimal performance and survival.

I thought of a similarity for all you Trekkie fans out there—remember the Borg? They were part-machine aliens whose mission was to ultimately overtake and subdue everyone they came in contact with; they would say, "Resistance is futile." Futile because the Borg would immediately adjust and assimilate itself to any type of resistance or aggression, making them nearly impossible to defeat. The body functions in a somewhat similar manner—whatever we throw at it, it fights back. Our immune system protects against diseases, antibodies fight germs, blood clots keep us from bleeding excessively, and our temperature protects the body core in extreme cold.

Now back to those scales. I saw a television sitcom once where the guy was so upset when his alarm clock went off he threw it out the window, only moments later having to search for it with a pair of binoculars to see what time it was. In like manner, I would fly into a rage and throw my scales into the garbage. Only afterward, I'd have to go out and buy another one. I guess I thought this new one would "say" what I wanted it to; kind of like, "Mirror, Mirror on the wall, who's the fairest of them all?" And it had better say me!

What you see however isn't always what you think you see. I have gotten up in the morning, looked in the mirror, and said, "I don't look *so* bad today." Then I'd step on the scales (usually after a near-starvation diet), and my weight either hadn't moved or would actually be up. I would become so depressed that even if I had looked like Bridget Bardot did in 1955, I'd *feel* like she looks now.

After getting older and wiser, I now realize that so many things are continually going on in my body making changes, adjustments, and also weight fluctuations. For instance, if you're putting on muscle, it weighs more; if you're not drinking enough fluids, your body will retain water; if you're in your monthly cycle, you always gain a few pounds. The *worst* thing you can do is get on those scales every day. I wouldn't even recommend it every week. If you must, once a month is sufficient to show a weight-loss trend, or to show you're maintaining your goal weight within a few pounds. The following advice will help to protect your fragile mind and ego:

*Never measure success by what the scales read.
*Always measure success by how your clothes fit.

Because there are so many factors influencing your weight, it doesn't always determine your actual shape or size. For instance, if you've added three pounds of muscle, and your weight is up a little, you probably look fabulous in a dress that three pounds fewer ago made you look pudgy. It's because your body has re-proportioned that weight.

We Have to Take Responsibility

Businesses are about making money. If we eat their food, and we continue to do it, we are in effect saying this is acceptable. If we want our lives back, we have to ultimately take responsibility for our health and commit ourselves daily to make the right choices. This isn't rocket science—just a commitment. We say we love this or we love that. The meaning of the word *love* is commitment. We make a commitment to God because we love Him and to our spouses because we love them and so on.

When we don't take care of ourselves, it's not just *us* we're hurting. I haven't really suffered alone all these years. My husband has been right there with me through thick and thin. I'm thankful for his commitment. You might be wondering, if this diet works where others fail—what's the catch?

If there's a catch, then I guess it would be that you won't lose ten pounds in a week like some weight-loss programs guarantee. My mind had always worked something like this: *"As soon as I lose this weight, I can't wait to go and get my favorite chocolate sundae and cheese burger!"* But there's nothing to go back to, like I chose to believe for so long. Your way of thinking has to change. When you see a cookie or cake, don't say, "Poor, pitiful me … I'll never have that stuff again." Instead say, "Tonight I'm having a big t-bone steak with a side of fries and stir-fry veggies!"

You need to forget that old destructive way of thinking and old way of life. This is an implementation of sound principles that will *make you* and *keep you* vibrant and strong. *Eat like this for the rest of your life.*

DIET Is a Four-Letter Word

At the mere mention that I might put my husband on a diet, he immediately becomes hostile and belligerent. He conjures up images of desperation, starvation, and depravation, to name a few. Give me a break! So I have to trick him by cutting out extra fat and calories and pretending it's the same ol' same ol'. Of course he tells me how wonderful everything tastes *until* I tell him it's fat free or 50 percent fewer calories than usual. Then he says, "I knew this didn't taste exactly right! You tricked me!"

If I allowed my husband to sit in his favorite chair with his remote in hand and eat all the bad, bad foods he loves, he'd die a happy man. And I do mean *die*. Of course you know I would never let that happen ... my next purchase: a cattle prod.

Chapter 10

Us Religious Folks

The Church

I would love to say we Christians have a lock on great health and good eating habits, but unfortunately sometimes I think we lead the pack in overeating. We have a covered-dish supper at the drop of a hat, and after a thirty-minute meeting, we'll serve up hot dogs with a table full of desserts to go along with them. I've heard a bunch of the brethren say, "We don't like finger foods." Well, it shows!

My brother accompanied me to a dinner theatre where they show a lot of religious entertainment, which naturally draws a lot of the church crowd. I told him to stay close behind me in the buffet line because people were likely to cut you off. After a couple of minutes, I happened to look back and I saw him far behind in line with a scowl on his face, he had been shoved out of the way and practically run over. Honestly we acted like hogs at the trough!

What Did I Eat Today?

1. I ate two big slices of whole-wheat pizza w/cheese, onions, peppers, and tomatoes.

2. Then I had a hamburger steak stir-fried with onions.

3. For a snack, I had a banana.

4. At supper I had a grilled chicken breast and small salad and a baked potato.

5. For a late snack, I'm eating mixed tropical fruit with fat-free whipped cream.

Notice: I had 2 proteins, 1 dairy, 1 potato, 2 fruits, 2 pieces of bread (whole wheat pizza crust), and unlimited green/salad vegetables, and my deliberate fat was in the pizza cheese. I used regular mozzarella instead of fat free.

What Would Jesus Eat?

The common acronym, "WWJD" which of course stands for "What would Jesus do?" inspired this section. Jesus is the only perfect man who ever lived, and he also had the perfect diet. He ate no processed foods at all. His diet consisted of whole grains, fresh fruits as well as high carbohydrate vegetables and high protein meats. He had a high-energy diet, which he needed because he walked everywhere he went (didn't drive a SUV).

Right now there are diet wars going on out there. Many doctors and scholars are saying the low-carb diets are the way to go, while other groups of doctors and nutritionists are saying high carbs are the way to go. And then you've got big weight-loss organizations with people who've lost over a hundred pounds. Some have indeed kept it off for quite a long time. However *statistically* the vast majority still gain their weight back and more (like myself). I have found over the years that whenever the Lord has given me a revelation of any kind, He has set the example for me already in his word.

The bottom line is this: Jesus is always right. When you want to know how to eat or how to do anything else, *look to Him*.

Chapter 11

Rhyme and Reason

Nutrition

Have you ever had several pieces of a puzzle, maybe a project at work or assembling something at home, but couldn't find that one piece that would finally pull it all together? Then one day, you find it, and it's like a light bulb coming on inside your brain. That's it! That's it! At long last, the mystery is solved.

If you don't remember anything else I say, remember this:

Nutrition is the key.

It's really the simplest thing, and yet it can be the hardest thing depending on your lifestyle and circumstances. Maybe you overeat out of boredom; or you may be subjected to a lot of junk food, so that's what you eat; or you might be like me—a food addict.

God designed our bodies to perform well in every way. But if you put trash in the gas tank of your car, it will sputter, stall, and eventually break down. In like manner, if you put trash in your body, it won't perform well either. But when you start feeding your body the high octane stuff, it will take off and start doing what it was designed to do: *Perform*.

The Quick-Fix Syndrome

We are the generation of the quick fix on everything. We're not willing to wait for anything or anybody, and we want it all and we want it *now*! For example, we will only buy cosmetics that claim to *instantly* erase our wrinkles or *instantly* make us look ten years younger. We want instant food, nothing from scratch (unless someone else cooks it). And we want instant job promotions and instant recognition for how wonderful we really are—I mean *we* see it, why doesn't everybody else?

And I concur. Remember I'm that fat, lazy American and have been most of my life. We live in an instant world, and *I like it*. I love to win. I hate to lose. Usually if I want something bad enough, I will give it all I've got. But I hate pain, so I always search for the easy way out. My motto: No pain ... no pain. That's why it's taken me thirty-three years of trying so many things to get myself together. Also, I'm no Einstein (as you've figured out by now). Here are two very important points to make:

You're never too old to learn.

You're never too old to achieve great success.

Some of God's greatest servants had their greatest success after they were getting along in years. Abraham and Sarah had a baby when they were nearly a hundred years old. Wow! Moses led the children of Israel out of Egypt in his eighties. Again, wow! And Miss Cynthia (that's me) was fifty-two when she finally listened to God and learned how to eat.

You know what? Sometimes I think you have to be older and more mature to be able to handle it. Maybe if I had been younger when success came, I might have thought I was "all that," but now I know I'm nothing apart from Jesus Christ and him crucified.

Now here's my third and most important point to make about the quick fix:

Wait on Jesus.

He's never late, and He's always right. Not everything comes to us quickly ... and sometimes, that's a good thing.

See ... I Told You!

As my weight has come off, everyone (especially women) have come up to me wanting to know my "secret." I told them I was working on a book that would be my personal story and what I did to finally win over weight. One day I was in a store in a large city trying on hats. I had started to tell several women who were discussing their weight problems about this book I was writing.

I had just begun to tell them about the diet when a young woman standing nearby spoke up and said, "I recently lost 170 pounds myself." We all turned to look at her (forget about me), and of course we all wanted to know how she did it. She said, "All I did was eliminate processed foods—mostly white flour, white sugar, white rice."

See ... I told you.

I'm Saying This for a Reason

I guess you wonder what I weigh. Let me say something before I tell you. Maybe for the first time ever, it's not really so much about my weight anymore and whether or not I wear a size 5, but it's about the overall quality of my life, how I feel, my new attitude, and yes, how I look. But invariably it's about taking my life back. Do you want your life back? Oh yeah, my weight. My highest was 195 pounds, and I was struggling on one of my harebrained diets (it's a wonder I had any hair or brains), when I realized I was going about this all wrong with the absolute wrong mindset and attitude.

Today I weigh around 142 pounds. My goal was 143. Being the consummate southern woman, I look forward to eating pan-fried corn, pinto beans (my favorite), and cashews. I wear mostly medium-sized garments, and because the weight has come off slow and steady, my skin isn't saggy or wrinkled. My husband and my girl friends all say I look great! But best of all—I'm happy with me. I'm *happy* ... and that says it all.

Chapter 12

Remembrances

An Inspiration

I sometimes think of the famous speech by Dr. Martin Luther King, Jr., when he exclaimed, "Free at last! Free at last!" with such passion and purpose. I don't dare equate myself with this great visionary, but I do finally understand freedom from a bondage that I've lived with most of my life, and other people continue to live with every day. It can eat away at your self-esteem, rob you of your happiness, and lessen the overall quality of your life.

When that victory that has eluded you for so long finally comes, you're able to understand how others feel who've had the courage to strive for something they believe in until they've achieved their goal. Freedom of the human spirit is a wonderful thing—worth living for, worth dying for, and worth fighting for.

That Girl

Some experiences stay with you—pleasant, beautiful, inspiring things you might see or hear over the years. I'll never forget a famous singer who once had one of the prettiest faces I'd ever seen. I always thought I wanted to look just like her. And then, (probably in her twenties) she started to gain a lot of weight, and that beauty started to slowly disappear. It was astonishing and very sad. I shall never forget her stunning beauty, and to this day I still look for her in the news to see if she ever lost that weight. I've never believed that being good-looking by itself would take you where you want to go in life, because it's who you are on the inside that gives you the drive to take yourself places. However it certainly doesn't hurt anything, and it *can* make the journey a little easier along the way in a beauty-oriented society.

Fat Synonyms

There was a woman I knew of a while back who had gained a lot of weight. Every time she spoke, I'd hear people saying cruel things like, "Did you hear that fat, ugly cow?" or "She's such a fat, stupid pig," or "If she'd get off her fat, lazy butt …"

Now why it is that "fat" seems to be synonymous with stupid, ugly, and lazy?

That same woman then lost a lot of weight, and she was one of the most beautiful women around. Keep in mind, she was the *same* person and she had the *same* personality. These former critics would now say things like, "Wasn't she funny?" and "Wasn't that sweet?" and "She's sooo cute!" Amazing, isn't it?

Chapter 13

Reactions

Celebrity Clause

There are diet books and exercise tapes for sale out there by many well-known celebrities. We react to them in a very positive manner because they're so successful and beautiful. Don't get me wrong—I applaud them, and I suppose this is their way of saying "do this" and "do that" to *continue* looking as wonderful as I do, and that's commendable. Most of the ones that come to mind, however, I've never known to be fat a day in their lives. I'm not talking about losing a few pounds to fit into a designer gown for the Academy Awards or exercising your way into a bikini for a photo shoot. Oh no!

I'm talking about a four-alarm, out-of-control situation that lasted for over thirty years!

The Strongest Statement Yet

It is unfortunate that overweight people are often treated badly. I've been there, and I know. But what I'm about to say is true, and it is the strongest statement I've made yet. It is this:

If you spend a million dollars on your wardrobe and have a cache of jewels to rival a queen, and if you have the best makeup artist in town, along with the best stylist in New York City—and you're fat … you might as well put a gold earring in a pig's snout!

Because *nothing* you put on and *nothing* you buy and *nothing* you do can ever take the place of the natural beauty God gave you. He created you; you're His handiwork, and all of those good looks are covered up with fat! Not to mention all the other things in your life covered up by this same fat—things like your self-esteem, your vitality, and your relationships.

Experience

You can have a PhD in everything from here to yon and an IQ of 200, but without experience, you're incomplete, because nothing takes the place of experience. When you apply for a job, what do all employers ask for?

My mother had nine children, and along life's way she encountered many difficulties (as you might imagine)—things such as life-threatening deliveries, illnesses, and financial setbacks to name a few. Many years ago, I went to see her because I thought I might be pregnant. She asked me when my last period was and about the circumstances surrounding it, then she said with supreme confidence, "Forget about it, you're not pregnant."

I said, "Are you *sure?*"

She replied, "I'm sure."

Over the years I've read prestigious articles and reports from highly credible and acclaimed professionals on various subjects of interest to me. But through it all, I usually acted on my mother's advice, who, without question or hesitation, gave me the right answer every time. How did she do it? Is she smarter than everyone else? Probably not. But she did have one thing so many others do not: she had experience. I'll never be as smart as my mother, but I do have thirty-three years of expertise in one area: food addiction and diets. This is one time *I* have the right answer.

Chapter 14

In Conclusion

It's Finally Over

I want this book to be different; I want it to be simple and to the point—exactly what I would want for myself. I want the truth, and I tell the truth, because I've been there and I know what I'm talking about. What would I like to see achieved from writing this book, you ask? I want to see choices out there in sandwich breads, pizza dough, rice, and sugar alternatives in all restaurants as well as supermarkets. But most of all, I want to see lives changed now and for eternity.

I would like everyone to be educated on what's making all of us, young and old alike, so unhealthy. We don't have to live this way. I want everyone to have a happy life. As 2 Corinthians 3:17 says, "[W]here the Spirit of the Lord is, there is liberty" (KJV). I've struggled for over thirty years, and I can tell you this: the next chocolate-chip cookie I eat will be in heaven, and folks, it won't be long—get ready!

If you have never received Jesus as your Savior, pray this simple prayer:

Dear Jesus, I believe you died for me and rose again. I ask you to forgive my sins and come into my heart and take over my life. Thank you, Lord, for giving me eternal life. I ask this prayer in Jesus's name. Amen.

My struggle is over ... it's finally over.

"Suffer not thy mouth to cause thy flesh to sin; neither say thou before the angel, that it was an error: wherefore should God be angry at thy voice, and destroy the work of thine hands?" (Eccles. 5:6)

Example of a Healthy Seven-Day Menu

Remember, this chart is only an example of how you might use your calories and fat each day.

Sunday	Monday	Tuesday	Wednesday	Thursday	Friday	Saturday
Buckwheat pancakes w/ pure maple syrup (fat)	Large whole-wheat bagel, cream cheese	Whole-grain cereal, skim milk	Cottage cheese, black cherries FF whipped cream	2 fried eggs, sliced tomatoes	2 slices of country ham, Fried apples	Yogurt w/ pineapple
Banana	Orange	Cantaloupe		Strawberries	Tangerine	Apple
Cottage cheese w/mixed fruit	Roast chicken, Steamed mixed vegetables	Turkey, green beans, potato (fat)	Low carb burger, baked potato	Whole-wheat pizza w/ cheese (fat)	Whole-wheat spaghetti, large green salad	Pork chops w/ teriyaki veggies (fat)
	Pear	Frozen mixed fruit	Banana sandwich(fat)	Tropical fruit	Glass of milk	
Steak w/ shrimp, baked potato	Baked fish, mashed potatoes, mixed greens (fat)	Japanese hibachi chicken w/mixed veggies	Grilled chicken salad w/ranch dressing	Roast beef w/carrots, onions, and potato	Pork BBQ w/ French fries (fat)	Chinese mushroom chicken

Many of these dishes are drive-through or carry-out meals from local restaurants. A lot of these burgers and ham you can pick up in a fast-food
drive-through window—so you do very little cooking.

You can pick up many of these items fresh daily in your local supermarket
deli.

Always keep microwaveable veggies and various fresh fruits on hand.

You can probably never completely eliminate all processed foods, especially when eating from restaurants and fast-food take-outs—but always
eliminate the forbidden whites from your diet, and you're over halfway
there!

Easy Grocery List and Health-Food Store Items

1. Sugar-free preserves

2. Brown rice—microwaveable

3. Vegetable medleys—microwaveable

4. Canned mixed fruit (in its own juice)

5. Fresh frozen mixed fruits

6. Roast (with carrots, onions, etc. for the crockpot)

7. Deli roast chicken, sliced turkey, etc.

8. Pure maple syrup (for wheat pancakes)

9. Skim milk, eggs, cottage cheese, yogurt, fat-free cream cheese

10. Fresh fruits of all kinds

11. Steaks, pork chops

12. Whole-wheat spaghetti and pastas

13. Whole-wheat flour

14. Natural sweeteners

15. Whole-wheat pizzas

16. Organic ketchup and other organic items

17. Various sugar-free drink mixes

978-0-595-43533-3
0-595-43533-5